THRIVING THROUGH THE UNEXPECTED

THRIVING THROUGH THE UNEXPECTED

FINDING HOPE IN DARK PLACES

LATRINA LENOIR

Published by *The Sunflower Circle Press*
October 2025

Thriving Through the Unexpected: Finding Hope in Dark Places

This is a work of nonfiction based on the author's personal experiences. Some names and identifying details may have been changed to protect individuals' privacy.

Published by *The Sunflower Circle Press* an imprint by Latrina Lenoir

For inquiries or permissions, contact:

info@latrinalenoir.com

Interior Design by Sohail Liaqat
Cover Photography Lauren Zoucha

ISBN: 979-8-9999075-0-9
Printed in the United States of America

DEDICATION

To my son;
You are the reason I breathe, the light in my darkest moments, and the heartbeat behind every word of this book. Your strength has been my anchor, your smile is my motivation, and your journey is the inspiration for my own healing.

To my daughter;
Thank you for your patience, your laughter, and your love. You have been a quiet strength in the background, and your presence reminded me that joy still exists even in hard seasons. You are a beautiful light in my life.

To my husband;
Thank you for standing beside me, even when the road was unclear and the weight was heavy. Your presence—even in silence—brought comfort. You held space for me while I was trying to find my way back to myself, and that matters more than you know.

To my father-in-law;
In the moments when I felt like I couldn't go on, you showed up. Whether it was staying overnight at the hospital, watching your grandson so I could catch a breath, or stepping in so I could finish school—your unwavering support carried me through. You didn't just help me survive; you helped shape the woman I am today.

To my grandmother;
I pray you are proud of the woman I've become. Thank you for pouring into me, for loving me unconditionally, and for raising me even after you had already raised your own children. Your sacrifices, your strength, and your unwavering love shaped the foundation of who I am. I wish you were here to witness it all. Everything I do—**it is for you.** I love you deeply and eternally.

To my cousin, Rosalind;
Thank you for cutting my son's hair when I didn't know how I would manage it. At the time, he had a movement disorder and was wheelchair-bound, and I wasn't sure any barber would have the patience for the task, but you didn't hesitate. I remember you telling me, *"Don't worry about it; I'll cut it for you."* And you did. You became his barber until he was able to sit still again for a haircut.

Thank you for watching him when I just needed a break—from being a mom, from being a caregiver. Thank you for being the listening ear I didn't even know I needed. Thank you for never judging me.

You played a major role in both my healing and Stephen's. Your kindness meant more to me than words could ever fully express.

To my therapist;
Thank you for the gentle but persistent pushes to return to writing. Though some chapters were more painful than others, it was through the writing process that I began to heal in places I didn't even know were still broken. Your guidance helped me put language to my pain, and purpose to my story.

To my close friends;
Thank you for the prayers, check-ins, shared tears, and moments of laughter when I needed them most. Your presence—near or far—reminded me that I was never alone.

And to every mother, father, caregiver, who has cried in the dark, felt forgotten, or wondered if you were enough—this book is for you. You are more than enough.

TABLE OF CONTENTS

PREFACE

My name is Latrina Lenoir, and I wear many hats; wife, mother, daughter, sister, friend, and nurse practitioner, just to name a few. Beneath all the titles, I am a woman who has weathered life's storms, clung to God's promises, and chosen to *thrive through the unexpected.*

This book was born from pain, but also from purpose.

Years ago, my world was turned upside down when my son—then a vibrant toddler—contracted the West Nile Virus just one month before his third birthday. What followed was a season of grief, confusion, and fear. Doctors told us he would never walk, talk, or eat again. But *God had the final say.* Today, he does all three. He is my miracle child—a living testimony of God's faithfulness.

The road hasn't been easy. My family has had to navigate challenges that many can't see from the outside. But through it all, we've experienced joy, healing, growth, and an unshakable hope that only comes from above.

In these pages, I open up about what it means to walk through dark places while still holding on to light. This isn't a fairytale; it's a faith walk. A testimony. A call to anyone who has ever wondered if they could make it through one more day. You can. And you will.

Thriving Through the Unexpected is for the mothers holding back tears in doctor's offices, for the caregivers who feel invisible, for the women who are pouring out while running on empty, and for anyone who needs a reminder that God still moves in impossible places.

You won't find perfection here. But you will find truth. Vulnerability. Laughter. Tears. And above all—*hope.*

So, take a deep breath. Settle in. Let me walk with you, friend. Not as an expert, but as someone who's been in the trenches and has lived to tell the story. A story of survival. A story of faith. A story of unexpected strength.

Welcome to *Thriving Through the Unexpected: Finding Hope in Dark Places.*

With love,

Latrina Lenoir

PART I

FOUNDATIONS OF MY JOURNEY

CHAPTER 1

I'VE EQUIPPED YOU WITH EVERYTHING YOU NEED

I've learned through experience that disability can strike any child or affect any family—at any time. On a summer day in May 2003, I left nursing school and picked up my healthy, active, soon-to be-three-year-old son from daycare. Little did I know, it would be the last time I'd see him that way.

Everything seemed normal—or so I thought. I arrived at the daycare, and there he was, my son, with a huge smile on his face, anticipating my arrival. He grabbed his things from the cubby, and we said our goodbyes to the staff. Our next stop was to pick up my daughter, who was about ten minutes away. I exited the car and went to get him out of his car seat. That's when I noticed it; a blank stare on his face. One I'd never seen before. I called his name several times but got no response. Seconds later, he began convulsing violently. I couldn't believe what I was witnessing. The ambulance was called and arrived within minutes.

We were taken to the nearest hospital. By the time we arrived, the convulsions had stopped but he was unconscious. He was breathing on his own, his heart was beating fine. No CPR was needed. We were told to wait for him to wake up. A CT scan and labs were done, but the results were inconclusive. When he did awaken, he was disoriented but calmed once he saw my face. After a few hours of observation, we were discharged with instructions to return if anything unusual occurred.

Still, my spirit wasn't settled. I returned to the daycare to ask questions; had he fallen? Hit his head? Anything? They assured me that nothing out of the ordinary had happened that day. I kept him home the next day just to watch over him. The evening was uneventful. The next morning, we followed our normal routine—breakfast, hygiene, and bath time for the kids. My children still bathed together at the time. Suddenly, I heard my daughter scream. Stephen was hitting her. This was odd for my usually passive son. I stepped in, told him to stop, and asked him to apologize. He did. But then, he stared at the bathroom light—the same blank gaze from before. I called his name. No response. I quickly grabbed him and placed him on my bed. Seconds later, he began to seize.

That wasn't his last seizure. They became more frequent, and he was eventually prescribed Depakote (an anti-seizure medication). Even though I gave the medication as prescribed, the seizures continued. I became exhausted with trying to keep up with school and his care. I spoke to my instructor and informed her of everything I was dealing with. I was carrying so much stress and exhaustion that I broke down in tears in my instructor's arms. I didn't know if I could continue living under so much stress.

My instructor allowed me to cry until I had no more tears. She sat me down and told me, "Latrina, don't worry. Go downstairs to the registrar's office and withdraw from the class for the semester."

I felt like a failure. I only had one test left to take (my final) before I completed the class requirements. But I knew deep in my soul-that something had to give; otherwise, I would have had a mental break down.

After I was able to gather myself; I proceeded to go downstairs to withdraw from the class. While I was walking, I felt like I was in a twilight zone. My legs were shaky and I was a bit slumped over. All I saw were bright lights as I walked through the halls. I couldn't focus on anything else around me; my mind was in a whirlwind. I wanted to finish nursing school, I didn't want to take a break or drop out, but I didn't have a choice. My son wasn't doing well on most days and I needed to be there for him. Nothing mattered more in that moment but taking care of my son. Still, there was this internal battle swirling inside me, telling me that I could do both, even though I wasn't coping by any means. With a myriad of thoughts running through my head on my way to the registrar's office, tears would stream down my face in the most unexpected moments.

Once I arrived at the window, I told the young lady what I was there for. I'm sure she could tell I had been crying. I could feel the puffiness of my eyelids. She didn't ask if I was okay or not, but she looked at me through the sincerest eyes. It was almost as if she hugged me without saying a word. After a few strokes on the computer, she handed me my paperwork back and confirmed my withdrawal from the class was successful. That moment lifted a huge weight off my shoulders. A weight I fully understood needed to be removed in that moment. I'd made the right choice.

There was one requirement after withdrawing from the class. I had to return to school before the Fall semester to take and pass my final exam. This would allow me to be promoted to my second year of nursing school.

Now that school was no longer stealing my time, I could focus on my children. I tried to keep my daughter's life as normal as possible, despite my world being turned upside down. This was truly a struggle. I would drop my daughter off at school in the morning and head straight to the hospital immediately after. By this time, my son was admitted to Loyola Hospital. The doctors were baffled because they couldn't figure out what was going on with my son. Test after test, results were coming back normal. But his body was telling us otherwise. I watched my son lose the ability to do the things he was able to do the day before. Within a week's time, my son lost the ability to walk, talk, or even eat on his own. He was basically a baby all over again. I was lost, devastated, and frustrated. I couldn't fathom what I was witnessing.

The doctors ordered more test. This time, they repeated the CT scan, an EEG, blood test, and a lumbar puncture (spinal tap). The repeat CT showed swelling of the brain, EEG showed progressive slowing of the brain waves, his white blood cell count was elevated, and the spinal tap revealed meningitis. He was started on antibiotics immediately while we waited to learn if it was bacterial or viral. If it was bacterial, we were working against time. Bacterial meningitis has to be treated quickly with antibiotics or it could be fatal. Viral meningitis is treated with supportive care (treat the symptoms), and allow it to run its course. After doing more definitive test, results revealed viral meningitis (West Nile). This was good news in a way.

He no longer needed antibiotics. But the virus was taking a toll on his tiny body. He was fighting hard, but in certain situations, I felt like the virus was winning. The virus caused his brain to swell rapidly and dangerously. On one occasion, a doctor said to me, "Mom, the next 24 hours are critical. We don't know if he will survive this or not. Only time will tell."

When the doctor left, I sat by the window, quietly crying, afraid this was it. Afraid that my son wouldn't make it. I didn't know what to do. I didn't know how to save my son. All I knew to do in that moment was pray and I honestly didn't know how to do that.

I didn't have a relationship with God at the time but I followed instinct. I just started talking to God like I was talking to a friend. The only thing I could say was, "God, please save my baby." The room was extremely quiet. I felt like I was in the eye of a tornado, quiet but in the path of possible destruction.

Seconds later, I heard a still small voice, "I've equipped you with everything you need."

I looked around to see where the voice was coming from. No one was in the room but me and my son. I trusted the voice. God had spoken. Hours later, Stephen's vital signs began to stabilize and the medications were finally working. The doctors did their rounds the next morning. They were happy with the stabilization of his vital signs and that his acuity level decreased slightly. We weren't out of the woods, but things were looking better.

Every day after, Stephen got better. After staying in the hospital for a month, we were finally discharged. My little boy, once so active and full of energy, could no longer walk, talk, or eat on his own. Our life became unrecognizable within 30 days. I left the hospital with a child that was now wheelchair bound, needed a feeding tube to eat, had a movement disorder, a TBI (traumatic brain injury), and a cognitive delay. I had no idea what my "new normal" would entail... But I would soon figure out this would be the start of one of the hardest seasons of my life.

During this time, I noticed that the visits from my son's father became less and less. It went from daily visits to weekly, biweekly, and then monthly—if we were lucky. There was really no explanation other than "I can't see my son like this." I was dying inside. I had no family there to support me. Some family members didn't come to the hospital because they said the hospital was too far. Others didn't give a reason; they just didn't come. My son's father was my only safe place at the time. When he withdrew, the only person who never left my side was my children's grandfather. His love and presence carried us through some of the hardest moments.

Through the pain, I found *purpose.* I was forced to make a decision. Either sink or swim. I chose the latter. God saved my son. So, I needed to step up and be all that Stephen needed and more. Was it hard? Absolutely!! I knew my baby needed me more than ever. He fought to live. Now it was my turn to fight to survive. I used his strength as my motivation to fight the battles I didn't see coming half the time.

The aftermath of our life was unpredictable, so this forced me to create a pretty structured life for the three of us. After life became more stable, I heard the same still voice that I'd heard in the hospital room; it was time to return to what I'd started. My children's grandfather agreed to watch them while I went back to nursing school. I felt comfortable enough where I could leave Stephen with him while I attended school. He knew how to administer the medications and feedings through the G-Tube. I taught him everything I knew, so that made things a little easier. Having his support, I not only returned to nursing school but also passed my final, the one I'd left behind almost a year earlier, with an A. I was so proud of myself.

I soon realized I hadn't ended up in nursing school by accident. I was strategically placed in a program that would become my son's and my lifeline. The more I studied, the more I asked questions. Based on the doctors' responses, I was able to make informed decisions. I became his nurse, advocate, and protector. After being discharged from the hospital, we'd attended intensive therapy (speech, OT, and PT) for 6 months. I never missed an appointment. His healing was my priority and now I was learning how to help him even more.

I was back in school but still unsure of what my future would look like. I'd made up my mind, though; I was there for a mission and I was intent on fulfilling it. My children deserved a better life and my son needed someone knowledgeable enough to articulate his health condition, understand and implement the necessary treatment modalities, and advocate to no end on his behalf. Though I was nervous about my return, I found a new group of classmates who became family. We supported one another emotionally, mentally, and spiritually.

We graduated with gratitude—and I did so with honors. We celebrated, passed our boards, and remained close. God's promise became my strength. His words stayed etched in my heart: **"I've equipped you with everything you need."**

Reflection:

Sometimes life hits before you feel ready.
But readiness isn't always a feeling—it's a truth God places inside of you. You may not always feel strong enough, wise enough, or brave enough. But God knew exactly what He was doing when He entrusted you with this journey. You don't have to have it all figured out. You just have to trust that what's *inside* of you is enough to face what's *in front* of you.

You've already been equipped.

Now walk in it.

Journal Prompt:

Think back to a moment in your life when everything felt like it was falling apart.
What helped you hold on during that time?
Was it a person, a word, a phrase, a scripture, or even an image?

Write it down. Revisit it. Let it remind you that you are stronger than you think.

CHAPTER 2

When No One Shows Up

There's a certain kind of grief that doesn't come from death; it comes from absence.

I felt it in hospital rooms filled with machines but empty familiar faces. I felt it when my phone didn't ring. When no one knocked on the door. When people who said they loved us were suddenly too busy, too far, too unsure. It's one thing to face a storm. It's another to face it alone.

I used to tell myself they didn't come because the hospital was far; although, public transportation was available 24/7. Or because they didn't know what to say. Even if they didn't say anything, their presence would've meant everything. Or maybe because it was easier to pretend everything was okay. But the truth is, when you're drowning, even silence can feel like betrayal.

I longed for someone to sit next to me and say, "This is hard. I see you. I'm not going anywhere." But they didn't. No one did. As a result, I learned to be my own cheerleader. My own rescue. I didn't grow up with a village that knew how to show up in hard moments. So, I carried that pattern into adulthood, hoping people would show up, and grieving quietly when they didn't.

Even now, I still wrestle with the ache. The ache of pouring out for others but rarely feeling poured into. But somewhere in the quiet, I realized something:

God doesn't abandon.

He sends who you need, even if it's just one person. For me, it was my children's grandfather. He showed up at the hospital when others disappeared. He stood in the gap, not just for Stephen, but for me as well. And sometimes one faithful person is more powerful than a hundred silent ones.

But even with him being there, the weight I carried didn't go away. I still felt like the entire world was on my shoulders. The doctor updates. The therapy appointments. Medication schedules. G-Tube feedings. The long nights. The constant wondering: *Am I doing enough? Am I a good mother? Will he survive? Will I survive?*

And through it all, the person who should've been standing beside me had chosen to walk away. It didn't feel fair that he got to escape: free to rebuild his life, laugh, sleep through the night, and move forward, while I was left holding all the broken pieces. How could he live so freely while we were drowning in the aftermath? How could he leave when we needed him the most? At our most vulnerable, when everything felt like it was collapsing, he disappeared.

The anger didn't fade; it grew. It rooted itself in my bones, especially during those moments when I had no choice but to keep going; no matter how exhausted or afraid I felt. His absence wasn't just physically; it was emotional abandonment, and it carved deep wounds I couldn't ignore. I wasn't just grieving the life we lost, I was also grieving the person who chose to not stay and fight with us.

I was so used to being the strong one, I didn't even know how to ask for help anymore. Truthfully, I didn't think anyone would come if I did. I had friends and family. But in this kind of battle, support means more than just checking in. It meant presence. It meant staying long enough to see the hard parts and not flinch.

Most didn't know what to say, so they said and did nothing. Others didn't know how to handle a little boy who could no longer walk or speak. But I did. Because I had no choice.

And somewhere in that loneliness, I started to realize something important for my survival: If you expect nothing, you won't be disappointed. That belief followed me for years. I became the one who did it all, all the time; partly out of strength, but also out of necessity and self-protection. I built walls where I needed bridges. I wore independence like armor, even when I was bleeding on the inside.

Caregiving will do that to you. It'll convince you that rest is a luxury, and asking for help is a weakness. It'll make you feel invisible. You will start to believe no one understands your life outside of you. They haven't survived a traumatic experience like this, so they likely will never understand.

And that's where the slow, silent grief begins; the grief of feeling unseen. The grief of holding everyone else together while wondering if anyone will ever hold you. **God reminded me that even in the absence of others, He had never left me.** I started talking to God like a friend—not with fancy prayers, just raw words, tear- soaked questions, and exhausted silence. He gave me peace that didn't make sense and strength I didn't know I had. He reminded me that being unseen by people didn't mean I was forgotten by Him.

It took time, but I stopped chasing support from those who didn't know how to give it. Instead, I started rooting myself in the One who saw it all—the late nights, the breakdowns, the quiet courage.

Looking back, I know now that God was training me, not just to survive, but to also walk in power. And strangely, a part of me had already been training my whole life.

Before I became a nurse, I became a mother. Before I ever walked the halls of a hospital wondering if my son would live; I grew up on the West Side of Chicago, where survival was a language, and strength was sewn into the fabric of every day. That place taught me how to keep going when everything in me wanted to quit.

It didn't teach me softness, but it did teach me stamina. And I would need every bit of that resilience for the battles ahead. Before I can tell you about our journey, I need to take you back to the city that raised me, the streets that tested me, and the family dynamics that shaped who I would become.

Reflection:

Some lessons are born in silence. Some strength is forged in solitude. You may not have had the support you needed, but you are still standing. That alone is proof that God's grace has carried you.

Journal Prompt:

Have you ever felt invisible in a hard season of your life?

What did that loneliness teach you?

Who, if anyone, surprised you by showing up?

Who do you still grieve that never showed up?

CHAPTER 3

GROWING UP IN CHI-CITY

Growing up in Chi-City had its ups and downs. Don't get me wrong—Chicago is one of the prettiest cities I've ever seen, especially downtown. The Mag Mile is breathtaking. The art, the culture, the energy—it's unmatched.

One of my favorite places was Navy Pier. You always knew you were near it when you spotted the giant Ferris wheel. The aroma of popcorn, hot dogs, and wings filled the air. Boat rides were to die for, especially on Wednesday and Saturday nights when fireworks lit up the sky. We'd catch the 8:30 PM ride to be on the lake when the show began. Afterward, we'd walk Michigan Ave and browse stores like Saks, Bloomingdale's, Neiman Marcus, and Coach. It felt like a world away from the crime, drugs, and danger we lived with daily.

On the West Side, life was different. We had fun, though, playing double dutch, hopscotch, and hide and seek just to name a few. Saturday mornings were my favorite. I'd watch *Saved by the Bell* on a tiny black-and-white TV in the kitchen. *Soul Train* followed. I'd dance along—stiff as ever, all while thinking I was the hottest thing smoking.

After the shows, I'd shower, dress, and head outside—never before noon per Grandma's rule. I was only allowed to stay on our block where she could see me from the window. Nick's store was across the street. I'd ask for $2 of spiced ham (cut medium), grab a bag of plain chips and an Orange Crush, then make a sandwich. That was a full-blown lunch to me! By nightfall, street lights came on and parents yelled our names out the window. We'd part ways by saying, "See you tomorrow."

Our home was crowded—six people in a two-bedroom apartment. My grandparents slept in one bedroom, my aunts and uncle slept in the other bedroom. There was a set of bunk beds and a full-sized bed in the second bedroom. I slept on the couch in the living room. At night, my grandmother would make me a pallet on the couch, and push a wooden table against the couch to keep me from falling off. She wasn't the affectionate type. I guess it was the way she was raised. I never got a hug or was told I love you, but I knew she loved me without a doubt. Her love was practical, not poetic.

She was my primary caretaker. My mom only picked me up on weekends. My mother became a widow when I was three years of age. My father left this world way too soon in his early 20s. He died of cancer and a brain tumor. After my dad died, my mother didn't seem as interested in motherhood as before. I'm sure his absence took a toll on her. They were high school sweethearts. Maybe life was too much to bear after he was gone. She started drinking heavily on the weekends. The weekends I spent with her were very chaotic—drinking, loud music, and often ended with me being disciplined with an electric cord. Welts on my body became a norm. It wasn't because I was being disrespectful or disobedient. It's because my opinion was different from hers, and when I tried to express my thoughts, it was taken as disrespectful. All under the guise of "a child needed to stay in a child's place." A child should only be seen and not heard.

I remember our apartment on Central Ave. We had metal bars on the doors, and on the weekends when I was there, Mom drank until she passed out. A neighbor, always concerned, checked on me when Grandma called him. He'd make me sandwiches and keep me safe.

At six years old, I didn't have the words for what I felt—but I knew the difference between chaos and safety. Grandma was safety. I just wanted to feel safe again. One weekend, fed up with the noise and confusion, I tried to sneak away and drive myself back to Grandma's. Yes, at only six years old. A stranger stopped me before I could start the car and got me home safely. When Grandma heard what happened from the neighbor, she came and got me. My grandma took two buses to get to my mother's. She used her extra set of keys to get in, got me dressed, and took me back home with her. My mother didn't have a clue what took place the night before—until she realized I was gone the next day. That Sunday, Mom called angry, but Grandma stood firm: "Why did you become a mother if you knew you weren't ready?"

I'm not sure what the response was on the other end of the phone, but my mother decided at that moment she wanted to be a full-time mother instead of part-time. She went to my elementary school and transferred me to the school near her home. She tried to play a full-time mom for a week. I could see the frustration on her face when she had to get me ready for school in the morning and comb my hair. She wasn't used to this. My grandmother had taken over the role since I was three. I hated the new school. I missed my friends terribly. After about a week, my mother was over it and I was back with Grandma—back to stability and safety.

My grandmother was the mother I was always searching for. I didn't have to look far. She was there the entire time. Even though I was loved by my grandmother, there was still a void that I wanted my mother to fill. I couldn't understand for the life of me why I was abandoned and rejected by her. In my six-year-old little mind, I thought I wasn't good enough. She didn't attend any parent teacher conferences, report card pickups, or any graduations (kindergarten, eighth grade, or high school).

What I didn't know at the time was that my mother was experiencing her own trauma. I was too young to understand. But God knew. He knew the void that my mother created was too large for her to fill. She didn't have the capacity to love me the way I needed her to. I often resented her for this. I often asked myself what was wrong with me. Did I look too much like my dad? Did I remind her of him? Did she hate him before he passed? She didn't speak much about him, but when she did, it was usually from a negative standpoint. What I learned later in life is that it was never about me—it was something within her that needed to be healed, so she could love her daughter unconditionally. Unfortunately, the healing never took place. We still have a strained relationship till this day.

Looking back now, I realize how much strength I carried in such a small body. Between the laughter of jump rope and the silence of locked doors, I learned how to survive. I learned how to hide pain behind jokes, how to care for others while craving love for myself, and how to dream of freedom before I even knew what freedom meant. It taught me how to stay quiet even when I wanted to scream. To smile so no one would ask if I was okay. That silence followed me for years.

My childhood wasn't perfect—but it was mine. And through it all, God was quietly equipping me for the storms I didn't yet know I'd face. When

I became a mother, I promised myself I'd be the safe place I didn't always have. I wouldn't be perfect, but I'd be present. And when life knocked the wind out of me years later, I would remember this little girl from the West Side who already knew how to keep breathing—even when the world around her didn't.

God had been whispering to me all along. I just didn't know it yet. But I'd need every whisper, every lesson, and every scar to carry me into the battle that was coming.

Chicago taught me how to survive. But it also taught me how to hide, especially when the pain became too personal, too shameful, too heavy to carry out loud. After years of learning how to bury pain behind smiles, I didn't realize I was walking into a season that would test everything I thought I knew about love, worth, and womanhood. I was still a child, but I was about to carry something much heavier than my age could bear.

Reflection:

Some of the strongest people were once little kids who carried too much. What you lived through shaped more than your personality, it also shaped your purpose.
You didn't just survive your childhood, you also outgrew it.
And you brought with you the kind of strength no book or classroom could ever teach.

Journal Prompt:

What's one childhood moment that taught you how to be strong, even if you didn't realize it back then?
How does that moment still echo in your life today?

CHAPTER 4

PREGNANT WITH PAIN, PUSHING THROUGH PURPOSE

Growing up in Chicago, we had a lot of fun as kids. We were truly raised by the village. Everyone in the neighborhood looked out for one another as well as the kids. We all played together until around the 7th or 8th grade. Families started to move out of the neighborhood because things were changing rapidly. More gangs and drugs began to infest the community. We saw more fancy cars with rims and gold chains than on TV. This was all so new and fascinating to us young girls who were barely making it. We dreamt about ways to become rich so we could become popular and wear all the stylish clothes and shoes. Little did we know, there was a dark side to the fast life. The most common paths that it led to was either jail or death.

As the environment began to change, so did I. I noticed more guys were paying attention to me, even though I was the girl who wore the ponytail to the side with a thousand scrunches. My shorts got tighter by the day. Not long after the neighborhood changed, a new family moved in. It was a pretty large family with a mixture of girls, women, and men. They dressed really nice and all the men had fancy cars with many gold chains around their necks. One of the girls ended up being in my class. We started hanging out after school. My grandmother didn't mind me hanging out with her because she lived across the street. She could come on the back porch to check on me. What my grandmother didn't know was that it gave me access to the boys she lived with, who were actually men. One of them showed interest in me and soon after, we found ourselves in a relationship.

I would soon find out he was 19 while I was merely 14. He already had a son. I believe he was a year old at the time. I found out when he and I were standing on the street corner talking and a young lady with a baby walked up. He began talking with her. He asked if he could be excused for a moment while he and the young lady walked away. This was red flag number one. He didn't introduce us. After a few minutes, he returned and I asked who the young lady was. He nonchalantly said, "Oh, that was my baby mama and son." I had the dumbest look on my face. Let's just say this was the precursor to many sleepless nights.

I was naïve to dating, so game was run on me Big Time. The cheating, emotional, and physical abuse brought my self-esteem way down. By this time, I started staying out late and my grandmother pretty much got tired of the lies. It was the summer after 8th grade graduation. She told my mom that she would have to raise me throughout my high school years. Well, that didn't last long. I ended up leaving my mother's house because I didn't want to babysit my life away. I was too busy being fast. By that time, I'd lost my virginity and started living with a friend. I pretty much lived with the boy and his mom. I dropped out of high school. I was just that in love (so I thought).

I was an Honor Student but I was willing to risk it all, even if that meant dropping out of school. I eventually got a job but didn't keep it because I partied all night and couldn't wake up in the morning. I was trying to be grown and have fun, but after a while, I started to realize this wasn't all it cracked up to be. I saw no future in my current situation. The guy I was dating was seeing several girls at the time, including me. Every day, it was a different girl. He would think I was in the house and he would drive different girls around almost every day of the week. When I would confront him, he would lie and want to fight me. According to him, the reason for fighting was because he was being faithful and I was accusing him of things he wasn't doing. Then, I would see the girls and ask them. Of course, they were happy to tell me that they were sleeping with him as well. Eventually, I got tired of the lies, cheating, and abuse. We went our separate ways and that was probably the best thing that happened to me. He had so many girls, it didn't faze him one bit.

After that chapter of my life closed, I began to feel happier and like myself again. I thought about enrolling back in school to get my High School Diploma. Through self-reflection, I knew better. I deserved better. I wanted more out of life. I had dreams and goals that I needed to fulfill. Why did I drop out of high school in the first place? If I stayed on track, the future ahead of me looked very promising. I'm sure I would've graduated with honors and attended a prestigious college. Why did I let lust get in the way of my purpose? I decided in that moment, I needed to enroll back in school and obtain my high school diploma. I wasn't allowing anything else to get in my way. Not a boy, love, or lust for that matter! I understood at that time; I needed to get out of my own way!

My saving grace, my grandmother, helped me enroll back in school. I was back on the right track, attending school regularly, and on the Honor

Roll. I wasn't able to attend "regular" high school because I wasn't in attendance for over a year, so I was required to attend an alternative school. It was good for me because I was around a new group of students without outside influence.

Reenrolling in school, there was another positive that I didn't have while attending my previous school. I was able to walk home. No more waiting on buses (especially in the winter time). My walk was about 15-20 minutes each way. One day while walking home on my way from school, I noticed a car following me. It was a familiar car but I couldn't tell who was driving it until it got closer.

Once the driver got closer, the car slowed down and the window rolled down. He asked, "Aren't you Christy's friend?"

I responded, "Yes."

He added, "I've been watching you for a while. You are growing up to be something nice."

I replied, "Thanks," with a smile.

He said, "Take my number and call me sometimes… You know, when you want to talk."

I was hesitant to take his number. One, I knew he messed around with my cousin before. Two, he was much older than me. Three, he wasn't the type of guy that I would usually date. And four, if I was going to be dating him, it would only be out of revenge. I was mad at my cousin at the time. There was a rumor around the neighborhood that my cousin messed with my ex-boyfriend, so I'd soon decide to "mess" with someone she dated. Later, I found out it was just a rumor. Once again, I felt like an idiot.

I took the phone number and put it in my dresser drawer where it stayed for a few months. Every now and then, I would see him and he would ask, “Do you still have my number?” I’d tell him yes, which I did. I just wasn’t interested in him at the time.

Well, one weekend, I went over to my aunt’s house. She was the cool aunt who would let her nieces and nephews drink alcohol and wouldn’t tell on us. She would even buy the liquor for us. She took me to the liquor store and purchased a drink named Cisco. It was a popular drink back then. Man, I got drunk so fast. I wasn’t a drinker and didn’t realize I was supposed to drink it slow. I drank it like it was pop. I’d taken the guy’s number with me to my aunt’s house. Once the liquor kicked in, I paged his beeper. He called back within five minutes. We had small talk due to the slurring of my words. I told him I would talk to him later on in the week.

I knew I would see him when I got back to the neighborhood on Monday. I couldn’t wait to get out of school so I could head home. I took my same path home and sure enough he pulled up alongside me. He asked me if he could take me home which was about a 5-7-minute ride. We chatted on the way and he dropped me off. This would go on for a few weeks before he asked if he could see me on a Friday night. I told him sure but I had an 11pm curfew. He was okay with that.

Friday came and he picked me up at 7pm. At first, we rode around sight-seeing and then we got something to eat at Sachels. I remember looking at the clock and it was 8:02pm. While looking out the window, I noticed we weren’t going back toward the neighborhood. We were driving westbound down Ogden. Next thing you know, we pulled up at Cindyland Hotel. He went in and paid for the room. At this point, I was scared because he was a full-grown man. I knew I wasn't prepared to do all the things grown men requested of me mentally or sexually. One thing led to another; little did I know this would be the beginning of a nightmare.

We still hung out with one another but he wanted me sexually in ways I just wasn't ready for. After I wasn't willing to do other sexual acts, he pretty much moved on to grown women instead of little girls like me. I couldn't blame him and didn't care. Well, about six weeks went by and my little friend didn't show up. My grandmother always had a saying, "When you sleep with older men, you get pregnant." I didn't want to believe I was pregnant. I took a home pregnancy test and sure enough two lines appeared on the test.

I was so sad and angry at myself. How could I be a fool yet again?

I kept it a secret as long as I could. My grandmother cooked breakfast and I stopped eating at the table. I would go in my room to eat because morning sickness was setting in. If I ate before noon, I was throwing up right after the meal. I knew I had to come clean. I called the baby's father and told him I needed to see him. He came and we talked. I told him I was pregnant and he responded, "Who are you pregnant by?"

I asked him, "Who else?"

He responded, "I was just asking… I needed to be sure."

I knew this news would break my grandmother's heart, and more than likely, I would be kicked out of the house. I told everyone on Christmas day. Everyone was opening their gifts and I told them I didn't have a tangible gift but I did have something to tell them. I told them I was pregnant. The disappointment I saw on their faces broke my heart. Not only was I not married, but I was also only 17 years old. They never met him because I knew he wasn't the one. It seemed like my stomach grew exponentially after breaking the news. It seemed like she was waiting on me to reveal the truth.

I didn't get put out but they didn't make things easier for me either. I still attended school and did what I had to do. I was determined to be a good mother despite my past mistakes. I enrolled into a school just for pregnant women. I did really well and remained focused. I didn't really hear from my daughter's father much after that. I would see him from time to time and we walked past one another like we didn't know each other.

A few months passed and I was getting off the Pulaski bus. He was on 13th and Pulaski. He saw me and he was mad at me. Till this day, I still don't know why. I think it may have been that the news got out about me carrying his child and he didn't want anyone to know. I got off the bus and he left his car running to walk toward me. He didn't utter a word. He grabbed me by the neck and shoved me really hard. I lost my balance and landed on my belly. I believe I was about 6-7 months pregnant at the time.

Although I fell, he didn't try to see if I was okay or anything. He got into his car, pulled off, and went about his business. I was in so much pain. The bus driver asked if I wanted him to call the police. I said no, but he called anyway. I went to the doctor and they couldn't find a heartbeat at first. The doctor called the ambulance and I was taken to the hospital for further evaluation. After a few minutes, they were able to detect fetal heart tones. I was kept overnight for observation. After being discharged, I stayed home. Luckily, school was out for the year and we were on summer break.

Eventually, I gave birth to a beautiful baby girl. Despite all I went through, I vowed to raise her with love, patience, and intention. I wasn't going to let my past define our future.

Reflection:

This chapter reminds me that healing doesn't happen all at once. It's a journey. I made mistakes, but I also made choices that changed the course of my life—for the better. My daughter became a light in a season that could've easily consumed me with darkness. I'm grateful that through pain, purpose can still be present. I'm grateful that through pain, purpose can still bloom.

Journal Prompt:

Reflect on a time when you were carrying something heavy—whether emotionally, physically, or spiritually—but still found the strength to keep going.

What "pain" have you carried that eventually revealed purpose?

How did that season shape your identity or shift your perspective?

If you could speak to your younger self in that moment, what would you say to her?

Write freely. There's power in honoring both the burden and the breakthrough.

____

____

PART II

ADVERSITY & AWAKENING

CHAPTER 5

SURVIVING THE PARK ROW HOTEL

Looking back, I realized some of the challenges I faced were the beginning of a much deeper lesson—one that would prepare me for the battles I didn't even know were coming. God was shaping something in me long before I became a mother. The lesson became a quiet strength that would carry me through a season of survival, testing my sense of safety, trust, and belonging.

That season began at the Park Row Hotel.

The Park Row Hotel was the hangout spot back in the day. Gangbangers, drug dealers, addicts, pimps, and prostitutes paid a visit to this place daily. The building sat on the corner of Roosevelt and Keeler, next door to the laundromat and across from the neighborhood food mart, Super Z. It wasn't your typical hotel. It was a four-story brick building, each floor housing 15-20 rooms.

The first floor was the busiest; traffic flowed in and out all day. The tavern, accessible from the main level, blared music that echoed through the halls.

It wasn't uncommon to walk past someone snorting coke in the stairwell or stumbling over people engaged in sex acts right in the hallway.

The second floor housed the kitchenettes. They were meant for single residents and a few struggling families. My mom and I lived in Room 219. It was small—one room with a bed, dresser, fridge, TV, and bathroom—but I never felt close to my mom. Although there was a bed, she made me sleep on a thin pallet on the filthy carpet. That carpet had seen years of life—hard, reckless life. It reeked of old beer, cigarettes, and something sour I couldn't name. The stains terrified me. Some were dark and crusted over; others were fresh and sticky. I would curl up tightly at night, trying not to touch too much of the floor, too scared to ask why I couldn't sleep on the bed. Our window looked out over the alley. During the day, it seemed quiet enough, but at night, it became something else. The sounds were unmistakable—moaning, cursing, car doors slamming, sometimes even shouting. I saw things no child should ever have to see. Sex acts happened constantly. Eventually, I stopped looking out the window altogether. I didn't understand it back then, but I knew it wasn't right. I knew I was too young to carry what those nights etched into my memory.

Most days, I was alone. My mom partied all night and stumbled home at dawn, reeking of alcohol. Sometimes, I'd already be awake, staring at the shadows from the alley moving across the walls. After she started leaving the window open, an unknown man began climbing through it at night. The room was dimly lit by the glow of the bathroom light—until he turned it off. He would approach me on the floor. My mother would scream and he'd flee. Still, she made me sleep there and make me keep the window up. I was just a child, but safety was never the priority.

I felt unsafe—physically, emotionally, and spiritually. But I had no choice. I still had to return there on weekends and during the summer so my grandmother could get a break. I was only 9 or 10, but I cleaned the room, stayed inside, and did what needed to be done while my mom vanished during the night.

During the week, I lived with my grandmother. Every afternoon after school, I carried dinner to my mom. My grandmother cooked for her Monday through Thursday. I also dragged our laundry across the lot every two weeks—heavy bags filled with clothes and detergent next door to the laundromat. My mom said I needed to learn how to take care of myself. I guess she was serious about that part.

One summer, everything shifted. My mom started sleeping more, eating more, and acting strange. Then she told me I had a sibling on the way. I remember thinking, *You can't even take care of me.* My grandmother was furious. When labor started, my mom dropped me off at Grandma's and went to the hospital. A few days later, she called to say she had a baby girl.

At first, I was excited. I loved my little sister. She felt soft, tiny, and like a real-life baby doll. But the excitement didn't last. My mom expected me to help raise her. Once my mom recovered, she was out again. During the week, my sister stayed with my mom, because I had school, so I couldn't be there all the time. Still, after class, I brought dinner and watched the baby.

One day, I used a key my mom gave me to drop off food. She wasn't there. I walked in and heard a strange gurgling sound. My sister was choking on a bottle that had been propped up. I panicked and grabbed her. I instinctively did what no one had taught me. Something that I remembered seeing on TV. I began to pat her back repeatedly. I just knew

I had to help her breathe. And when she finally did, when that cry pierced the silence of the room, I exhaled a breath I hadn't realized I was holding.

When my mom returned, she didn't ask what happened; she blamed me. And then came the discipline. I didn't even try to explain. What would've been the point? I had saved her life, and somehow, I was still the problem.

That moment shook something loose in me. I wanted to be there for my sister but I never wanted to go to my mother's house again. All I'd ever done was go there —to do the laundry, to bring her food, to look after my sister—and all it came with was blame for one thing or another. Still, I kept showing up. Even when I didn't want to. Not out of obedience, but out of fear—fear that something might happen to my sister again, and this time no one would be there to help her.

That day taught me how to listen for silence. To hear the danger in quiet rooms. I learned how to be calm under pressure before I even understood what pressure was. I didn't know it then, but I was being trained—for my daughter, for Stephen, for a life that would demand both tenderness and strength.

When I became a mother, I didn't flinch at midnight cries or emergencies. I already knew how to stay when it was hard. I already knew what it meant to carry someone else's breath in your hands.

Looking back, I think that moment was the first time I ever felt the weight of responsibility—and the sting of injustice. But it also marked the beginning of a deeper strength, one I'd call on again and again in hospital rooms, therapy sessions, and long nights sitting on bathroom floors holding my children through tears.

And maybe that's why my sister clung to me—not just out of love, but because I had always shown up. I had always reached for her when no one else did. I was her constant. Her safe place. And despite everything, I wouldn't have it any other way.

Because that day didn't just teach me how to save her, it also taught me how to **be** a safe place. And that would become the legacy I carried into motherhood; *to be what I never had.*

Reflection:

Sometimes the most dangerous places aren't just physical—they're emotional landscapes where you're forced to grow up too fast. I didn't have a choice but to become responsible, alert, and mature before my time. I cleaned up after adults, cared for my baby sister, and watched over a mother who rarely watched over me.

The Park Row Hotel wasn't just a building; it was a symbol of abandonment, survival, and silent prayers whispered on dirty floors. It taught me how to function in dysfunction, how to protect others even when I wasn't protected, and how to listen for God's voice when the world around me was too loud to hear anything else.

And yet... I made it.

The child who once lay frightened on that stained carpet eventually stood up, learned her worth, and refused to carry shame that was never hers to bear.

Journal Prompt:

Think back to a time when you had to grow up too soon.
Maybe you were forced to take on adult responsibilities as a child. Maybe you were left to figure out safety, love, or survival on your own.

- What did you learn to carry that wasn't yours to carry?
- In what ways did you protect others while still longing to be protected yourself?
- How did that experience shape your beliefs about trust, love, or your own worth?
- If you could sit with your younger self in that moment, what would you tell her?

Let this be a safe place to pour out what you've held in for far too long.

CHAPTER 6

What Looked Like Loss Was Love in Disguise

I met my son's father during a time when I least expected it; while I was pregnant with my daughter.

We were introduced through mutual friends. His cousin was dating one of my friends, and we often hung out in the projects together. He'd offer to drive me home afterward, never asking for gas money, never trying to flirt, or even ask for my number. Honestly, I was relieved. I was already pregnant by someone else, and the last thing I needed was another layer of complication.

But he was kind. Gentle. Always pleasant.
He said yes to anything I asked, even when he didn't have to. He made sure I got home safely, every time. And though I tried not to entertain it, there were moments when I wondered what it might be like to be with someone like him. Someone steady. But then I'd remind myself; *I'm carrying another man's child.* I assumed he'd never want to take on that kind of responsibility. At the time, he didn't have any children of his own.

A few months passed, and I gave birth to a beautiful baby girl. I stayed home during those first precious weeks, wrapped in new-mom life until I was cleared to get out again. When I finally did, I caught a cab to see my friends. I needed a little girl time—a breath of normalcy.

The hours flew by, and before I knew it, night had fallen. I was gathering my things to call another cab when he offered to drive my daughter and me home. That one ride turned into many with the three of us. Still, he never asked for my number—and I couldn't help but wonder: *Maybe he has a girlfriend?*

I started coming around more, but I never saw him with anyone. Over time, our exchanges grew into conversations. We started joking, laughing, teasing. Something gentle was forming between us. A quiet closeness.

One day, my phone rang. It was my friend from the projects, laughing so hard she could barely speak.

"Girl," she said between giggles, "Steve is over here talking about he had a dream about you!"

I paused, confused. *Wait, what?* Was I hearing that right?

My heart skipped.

While slightly smiling, I asked to speak to him. He got on the phone, and I asked, "So…you had a dream about me?"
Without hesitation, he answered, "Yes."
Then he handed the phone back to my friend like it was nothing.

I laughed. "I'm going to get the baby dressed," I told her. "I'm heading over there."

When I arrived, everyone was laughing, like it was some inside joke I had just walked in on. I looked at him and asked, "So, you had a dream about me? What was it about?"

He smiled. "Yeah, I did."

But he never told me what it was about.

Instead, he asked me to step out on the porch so we could talk in private. I agreed and went with him. I can't quite remember how the conversation went; it's a blur now. What I do remember is the feeling that something real had just begun.

That moment was the start of what would become the building blocks of our relationship. From that day forward, we started spending more and more time together. What made me fall in love with him wasn't just how he treated me, but also how he cared for my daughter.

I was a true mama bear—protective and particular. But he was more curious, more invested, more hands-on than I was at times. He'd ask questions like: How do you make the bottle? How do I change her clothes? What if she spits up; what should I do?

He wasn't like the guys I had known before. He was different. Gentle. Intentional. Present.

He celebrated every milestone as if she were his own—her first solid food, her first tooth, her first steps. He carried her like she was something priceless. And when she cried, he picked her up without hesitation.

She wasn't his biologically, but in every other way, she was his daughter. That's when I knew I'd had a baby by the wrong man.

He showed me what fatherhood could look like. Something I had never seen growing up. My own father died when I was just three years old. I have no memory of him. But watching my boyfriend with my daughter…it was like he was laying down a blueprint for me. Showing me what love could look like in action.

I was on a high from life. It felt too good to be real. And sometimes, it was.

We'd break up, find our way back to each other, try again, fall apart—and try again.

But then came the argument that changed everything.

It started like any disagreement, but this time, the tension didn't settle. It exploded. We both said things we couldn't take back, and instead of making up like we usually did, we walked away.

What followed was a silence that lasted a little over a year.

That breakup was painful. Not just because we were apart, but because so much was left unresolved. I had gotten used to him being there—not just for me, but for my daughter as well. And now I was navigating life alone again, pretending I was okay when deep down I felt the void. I missed his presence, his steadiness, the way he lit up when she smiled. I didn't know if we'd ever find our way back.

But somehow…we did.

Our paths crossed again, and something in us had shifted. The love hadn't disappeared; it had been waiting, growing, maturing. We approached each other differently this time. With more humility. More listening. More grace.

Eventually, we decided to give it another real try. By then, my daughter was two and getting ready to start daycare. She thought he was her father—and in every way that mattered, he was. Her biological father had been mostly absent. And as much as that used to hurt, I came to see it for what it was: a blessing in disguise.

I wanted the situation with my daughter's father to be the blueprint of what not to do/choose in another man. For this reason, I wanted to learn everything about how men were wired so I wouldn't end up in the same situation twice. A single mom without a present and caring father for her child.

Overtime, I would hear older women say, "The way to a man's heart is through his stomach." So, one day while grocery shopping, I picked up a box of Hamburger Helper. I read the instructions right there in the store, bought the ingredients, and decided to give it a try. I even added garlic bread.

That was the first meal I'd ever cooked completely on my own. Growing up, the girls in our family weren't allowed in the kitchen. We had to figure it out ourselves.

It wasn't gourmet, but it was made with love. My boyfriend devoured it and asked for seconds. Even my daughter loved it. At that moment, it felt like we were becoming a real family.

Everything seemed to be falling in place again. But there was always a reminder in the back of my mind; I had a child with someone else. Every now and then I would run into my daughter's biological father in the neighborhood when I went to visit my grandparents. This particular time I saw him right before Christmas. A few weeks earlier, I went Christmas shopping and had a layaway of clothes for her. The balance was just $60. I asked if he could help cover it. I planned to pay it off myself if needed, but it would've been nice for him to contribute.

He finally gave me the money—but not without a comment: "Don't go get your hair done with this," he said.

I was stunned. "Even if I did," I told him, "that still wouldn't come close to what I've spent raising her on my own." To be fair, after I picked up the clothes, I called him to let him know. And that was the end of it.

Sometimes we think God takes people away to punish us. But it's not punishment—it's protection. God was clearing space for something better, someone better.

My daughter's life has been abundant—not because of what she lacked, but because of who stepped in and stayed. My boyfriend (now husband) loved her like she was his own. He showed me what fatherhood could look like. And in doing so, he began healing parts of me I didn't know were broken.

After a few years of dating, I became pregnant with our son.

We were in true bliss.

Right around that time, a two-bedroom apartment opened up downstairs in my building. It was perfect. I had just finished a college semester and was planning to take the summer off to prepare for baby number two.

Shortly after giving birth, my sweet neighbor knocked on the door. She'd noticed she hadn't seen me in a while and figured I had delivered. She asked to see the baby, and instantly fell in love with him.

That woman became our lifeline. We called her **Dimples.** She babysat for us so I could return to school and work. She loved my kids like they were her own. When she eventually moved to another neighborhood, she offered to keep them but the distance was too far. I didn't have a car, and it broke my heart to lose her daily support.

To this day, I wonder where she is. I wish I could thank her again for all she did for us. She was an angel in disguise.

Reflection:

Sometimes, the detours in life—the unexpected moves, the hard transitions—are divine setups. What feels like a loss may actually be love in disguise. Keep your heart open. Help can come from the most unexpected people at just the right time.

Journal Prompt:

Think back to a time in your life when something you desperately wanted didn't work out—maybe a place to live, a job, a relationship, or a dream. At the time, it may have felt like a painful setback.
Looking back now...

- What did that loss feel like in the moment?
- How did that situation help you grow or protect you?

- Is there something or someone you now see differently because of what you went through?

Write about how your perspective has changed—and how loss may have made room for something greater.

CHAPTER 7

MOTHERING THROUGH GUILT AND GRACE

Just when I thought the hardest battles were behind me, a new one emerged. Not with doctors, not with diagnosis, but with someone I never expected; my daughter. I noticed subtle changes once I brought her brother home from the hospital. I was overwhelmed. I didn't have much help.

I was so scared I brought him home to die. There were many nights I would lay there and watch his limp body lay across my bed. His chest would rise and fall, giving me small glimpses of hope. I was trying to prevent one child from dying, while the other child was still alive but dying inside. She needed consistent attention, love, and hugs. What she needed most was her MAMA.

As hard as it is to admit, I failed her. Not because I wanted to, but because I had no choice. The resentment started as a small brick until it eventually became a boulder. I didn't love her any less. I was trying to be the best mother I knew how to be. In her eyes, that wasn't enough. She was too young to understand. She didn't know I was only staying alive because of them. I wanted to die every day I opened my eyes and had to relive my new normal again.

I fell into a deep depression, but nobody knew. I smiled and acted as if everything was okay, but I was really dying inside. I didn't eat much because I just didn't have an appetite. The weight started to fall off. If someone would've asked me how I was, I wouldn't have known the answer because I really didn't know. Only one thing I knew for sure: I LOVED MY KIDS WITH EVERYTHING IN ME!! Loving my daughter has been one of the greatest honors of my life, but it has also exposed the deepest cracks in my heart!

How do you carry both grief and guilt and still try to show up whole? She felt abandoned, rejected, isolated, sad, and angry with life. I couldn't blame her. I felt the same way. I often asked myself: why would a good God allow this to happen to my child? To us? Why me? Would I ever be able to mend my relationship with my daughter? Will she forgive me? Would she understand the sacrifices I made for them? Will she still love me as her mother or find a mother figure to take my place?

There were many times my daughter would rather be around her godmother than me—and truthfully, I understood why. As her brother aged, the more care he required. She hated me because of this. It came to a point where she was no longer interested in what I had to say. I was angry with her and God. I didn't ask for any of this, but yet I rose to the assignment with grit and grace. I knew we could've lost him, but she didn't care. As my daughter got older, we butted heads so often that at one point, I thought it would be better if her godmother raised her. I didn't have the conflict resolution skills I have now, and looking back, I wish I would've fought harder for our relationship.

Every special moment felt like it came with tension. One of the hardest moments for me was on my wedding day. What was supposed to be a celebration turned into a memory tainted by her behavior. I couldn't understand how someone I loved could choose that moment to act out. But now, with time and healing, I realize hurt people often hurt others, especially when they don't know how to express their pain. One year, she took me out for Mother's Day, only to later say I cost too much. She picked the location and planned the whole thing. I was stunned.

At times, I feel like I'm trying to love her through a wall of resentment. It's a wall I didn't intentionally build, but it's there—brick by brick, formed by misunderstandings, unspoken expectations, and emotional wounds on both sides. She feels like I love her brother more. Even as adults, this narrative continues to shape our interactions.

The truth is, I've had to parent two children in drastically different ways. One child required around-the-clock care due to a life-altering illness. My attention was often split, and I know now that she experienced that as rejection. That wasn't my heart, but it was her reality—and I have to honor that truth.

If I could go back, I'd choose more softness, more presence, more patience. I'd hold space for her feelings instead of trying to "fix" them. I would've told her more often: *You matter just as much. I see you. I love you.*

We're still healing. We still have difficult conversations. But I believe in reconciliation. I believe in grace. And I believe that while wounds can run deep, love can go deeper.

Reflection:

Have you ever loved someone through unresolved pain? Are there parts of your parenting journey you wish you could revisit with the wisdom you hold now? Take a moment to sit with those feelings—not in shame, but in awareness. Healing begins when we stop hiding our hurt and start giving it a voice. Let love lead the way.

Journal Prompt:

What unspoken emotions have shaped your relationship with your children or loved ones? If you could write them a letter today, what would you say?

CHAPTER 8

SIBLING RIVALRY – HEALING THE UNSPOKEN WOUNDS

My sister and I didn't grow up in the same household. I was raised by my grandmother and she was raised by our mother. That alone created a rift we never truly understood until much later in life.

Our separate upbringings exposed us to different versions of love, discipline, and stability. I had structure; she had unpredictability. And though we were both doing our best to survive what we were handed, we developed very different tools to cope. Instead of those tools helping us connect, they often clashed.

We bumped heads more often than we embraced. Conversations turned into arguments. And when we were in the same space, it felt like there was an invisible wall—one neither of us knew how to break down. Behind the smiles at family events were buried disappointments and the ache of not knowing how to simply be sisters.

Maybe this is due to our upbringing. Perhaps outside influences. There were many variables that played a part in our distance. I always tried to be the best big sister I knew how to be. I showed up with love, hugs, and whatever else was required of me.

But the sisterly love wasn't always reciprocal. And that broke my heart.

I often thought to myself, *How is this possible? It's only two of us. We need each other. It's supposed to be us against the world.* Unfortunately, I was the only one who felt that way.

There were times when we didn't speak for years. In fact, at the time of writing this book, it has been three years since we've last spoken. Not because of something we did to each other, but because she allowed an outside force to come between us. I begged her not to let it happen, I even explained why, but my words didn't matter.

As the years passed, the wounds didn't fade. They festered—silently. There were moments I wanted to draw close, but didn't know how. And I'm sure she felt the same. Sometimes she'd choose others over me, and I would do the same. The divide wasn't about hate—it was about hurt.

But the hurt got heavier when life got harder.

When my son fell ill and our world turned upside down, I needed her. Not just emotionally—but physically, mentally, and spiritually. I was overwhelmed. Fighting for his life. Barely sleeping. Barely breathing. I was stretched beyond what any mother should ever have to endure.

I thought, surely, if there was ever a time she would show up it would be then.

But she wasn't there.

There were days when I was drowning in caregiving—changing diapers, administering medications, watching my son's chest to make sure he was still breathing—and all I wanted was someone to knock on the door and say, "I've got you." I didn't need perfect words. I just needed presence. I needed *her* presence.

I remember holding my son in the middle of the night, praying he'd make it through until morning. And in the next room, my daughter was quietly falling apart. I was split between two impossible needs. And there were moments I just needed someone to be there for *me*—to let me cry, or sleep, or breathe. My sister never came.

I tried to extend grace. I tried to assume the best. Maybe she didn't know how to show up. Maybe her own pain kept her away. But that didn't erase how deeply I wished she'd come. That absence left a mark.

I resented her—for celebrating life while I was holding mine together with prayer and pure willpower. For being silent during the storm.

And that silence…it was louder than anything she could have said.

I never expected her to fix it all. I didn't expect perfection. I didn't need her to rescue me. But I did expect *compassion.* I longed for grace from her. Not judgment. Not distance. Just grace. The kind I would've given her without hesitation.

That unmet hope changed me. It hardened me in some places and softened me in others. It taught me to release expectations—even the ones that felt basic, even the ones I thought I was entitled to. It taught me how to keep loving someone who couldn't or wouldn't show up the way I needed.

There's something unspeakably painful about needing someone during your darkest hour and realizing they won't come. Not because they're gone, but because they chose not to. And yet—somewhere deep inside—I still loved her. I still do.

There were pivotal moments—birthdays, weddings, holidays—when our tension surfaced in ways that left lasting impressions. Looking back, I can now see how much of our conflict was unspoken pain. I was angry at the brokenness and so was she. But neither of us had the language or emotional tools to say, "I miss you," or, "This hurts."

Healing hasn't come yet but I have hope that it will. If she ever reads this book, my message to her would be: We weren't ever meant to be enemies. We were just two little girls trying to survive different storms. I hope one day you will see me not through the lens of old wounds or misunderstandings, but for who I truly am. I hope you know that you have always been and still are loved deeply by me. No matter how far apart life may take us—even if we never speak again—that truth will never change.

Reflection:

Not all relationships find resolution in a neat bow. Some need space. Some need time. And some simply need truth. Sibling relationships can carry generations of misunderstanding and unmet needs, often hidden beneath silence. Healing may not always mean reconciliation—but it can still mean peace. It begins with acknowledging your truth without shame, and theirs without judgment.

Journal Prompt:

- What part of your sibling relationship still feels unresolved?
- What do you need to release in order to begin healing, even if nothing changes on their end?
- How have your childhood experiences shaped the way you show up in relationships today?

PART III

FAITH, HEALING, & BECOMING

CHAPTER 9

THEY SHOWED UP WHEN IT MATTERED

Growing up on the West Side of Chicago had its pros and cons. One of the biggest pros? The incredible neighborhood role models who shaped my early years. At Matthew A. Henson Elementary School—the Henson Hornets—the staff genuinely cared about us. They weren't there just for a paycheck. They took pride in teaching and they believed in our potential.

Mr. Williams taught 7th and 8th grade. His voice echoed from the third floor all the way down to the first. He could teach any subject, but music was his passion. During assemblies or graduation performances, his class always brought the heat! He worked us hard but made us better. When frustrated, he'd take a smoke break, then come back calm again.

Ms. Ott, the 7th-grade teacher, was all business. She wore skirts every day and had a no-nonsense attitude. I acted up in her class, until I learned she lived near my mom. Small world! Her nephew was my friend, and we silently agreed to keep each other's secrets.

Mr. White, the gym teacher, was legendary. We cried if we missed gym. He taught us discipline, teamwork, and how to push ourselves. And yes—he had a paddle! He kept many boys out of trouble and inspired them to be men. May he rest in peace.

Mr. Cockrell was our school security guard and basketball coach. When I was teased for wearing Payless shoes, I cried my way to the office. I was so embarrassed. Kids can be cruel and they knew the shoes came from Payless. I remember staring at the floor trying to disappear as they laughed.

I didn't tell anyone how much that situation hurt me. But Mr. Cockrell noticed. Mr. Cockrell saw me and asked what was wrong. At first, he couldn't understand me due to ugly crying. He sat me down at his desk that was positioned in the corner across from the main office. He allowed me to calm down no matter how much time it took. He was patient. He cared. After about 10 minutes, I told him what happened. You could tell by the expression on his face that he was angry. I was a good kid and didn't bother anyone. I didn't tease kids because I knew what it was like to live in lack. I didn't have all the latest clothes or shoes but I was clean and clothed prior to leaving my home.

The situation must've really bothered Mr. Cockrell. Later that week, he took me to get my first pair of name-brand shoes—blue and white Bo Jacksons. His act of kindness wasn't just about the shoes; it was the first time I felt like someone saw me and said, "You deserve more." When I laced up those Bo Jacksons, I stood a little taller. Not because they were name brand, but because someone believed I was worth it. I was thrilled. But some of my family members weren't. They believed in suffering in silence. I was told never to accept help from outsiders. I share these memories not to call out the hard parts, but to spotlight the people who poured into me when I needed it most. So today, publicly: THANK YOU, Mr. Cockrell. You changed my life.

Lastly, Kina Montgomery—my nursing instructor, my mentor, and someone who once held a very special place in my life. She poured into me during a critical season. She taught me how to think critically on my feet, how to care for others with both compassion and confidence, and how to believe in myself even when I felt like giving up. She helped me raise my daughter when I was overwhelmed, taught me how to cook, supported my dreams, and encouraged me to pursue becoming a nurse practitioner. Her presence was a gift I will always be grateful for.

I remember one day, one of the students in my class called to check on me. She wanted to see how I was doing after I withdrew from the program. I couldn't take it anymore. Trying to be strong was breaking me inside. I burst into tears: "I'm not doing well. Stephen keeps vomiting after every G-Tube feeding. I'm afraid he is going to end up back in the hospital due to dehydration and malnutrition." I sobbed on the phone and uttered, "I have done everything. I don't know what else to do."

About an hour later, I got a phone call from Kina (my nursing instructor, who later became my daughter's godmother). She explained to me that he wasn't digesting the food. I needed to space his feedings out longer. She told me to check the residuals (aspirate stomach contents) two hours after the feeding. If the residual was more than 60 ml, I should check again in an hour. If it was less than 60 ml, it was okay to restart the feeding. After that call, Stephen never vomited again. I started doing exactly what she'd said and he began gaining weight and started to look healthier.

The discharge instructions from the hospital didn't include this pertinent information, or maybe it did. I was so overwhelmed with so much information that I didn't know if I was coming or going. Looking back, a home health nurse for a week or two after discharge would've helped tremendously. Kina didn't just teach nursing, she modeled it. She gave grace when I had none left for myself. That kind of mentorship changes you for the better. I'm forever grateful for the role she played in our lives. God used an ordinary person to plant extraordinary hope in my heart. And I held on to that hope for dear life, especially when life got hard again.

Though our paths have since gone in different directions, and our relationship is no longer what it once was, I still honor the impact she had on my life. Some people are meant for a season, and Kina's season in my life was filled with purpose, growth, and invaluable lessons. I will never stop thanking God for the way she helped shape the woman I am today.

Reflection:

Sometimes, the people who impact us the most aren't related to us by blood; they're earthly angels placed in our path to guide and uplift us. Their lessons, love, and presence leave lasting impressions. To all the role models who shaped me: Thank You!!

Journal Prompt:

Think about the people in your life who showed up for you during a difficult season—big or small.

- Who are the people that made you feel seen, supported, or safe?
- What did their presence mean to you in that moment?

- Have you ever been that person for someone else? What did it feel like?

Take a few moments to write a letter (even if you never send it) to someone who showed up when you needed it most. Let your gratitude flow.

CHAPTER 10

THE POWER OF SELF-CARE

For years, I wore my strength like an armor. I believed that being strong meant pushing through exhaustion, saying yes when I should've said no, and putting myself last on every list. I thought self-care was selfish—something reserved for people with time, money, or fewer responsibilities. But eventually, I learned a powerful truth: **Self-care is survival**.

As a wife, mother, caregiver, nurse practitioner, and advocate, I spent so much time tending to the needs of others that I barely recognized the woman in the mirror. My energy was depleted. My joy felt distant. And my body was waving red flags I could no longer ignore. It wasn't until I hit a breaking point that I realized something had to change—not just for me, but for the people who depended on me.

There were seasons I operated on fumes—navigating hospital stays, therapy appointments, work demands, and emotional breakdowns without pause. I told myself I was strong, but deep down, I was crumbling. I remember sitting in my car outside of the clinic one day, watching other people walk in with their loved ones while my son was barely hanging on.

I was numb. I was frustrated. I was angry that God allowed this to happen to my family. I had been up for 36 hours. I hadn't eaten. I had no one to call.

I laid my head on the steering wheel. The horn was blowing. I didn't care. I gripped that steering wheel for dear life. My knuckles turned white due to how hard I was gripping. I burst out in tears and wondered: *God, how much longer? Haven't I been punished enough? Is he going to get better?* I sobbed like my son's next breath depended on it. I was breaking from the inside, not because I was weak, but because I had been too strong for too long.

After what felt like a lifetime—which in reality was about 2-3 minutes—I lifted my head to look ahead. There were people staring. They had concerned looks on their faces. They wondered if I was okay. I let my window down slowly, and through the tears that filled my eyes, let them know I was okay; I was just having a moment. I could taste the saltiness of my tears on my lips.

My son was in the back seat crying as well. He wasn't crying because I was crying. He cried because I startled him with the noise. The horn that blew continuously for 2-3 minutes. I quickly apologized to him. He had been through enough trauma and I didn't want to add to it. He calmed down after I rubbed his head. I wiped his tears and he was back at ease. Once he calmed down, I realized I needed to do the same thing for myself.

I took really deep breaths, one after another. After 20 minutes, I was calm enough to take my son to his appointment. I got a good report that day. Stephen was able to track objects with his eyes. That was huge relief. The doctors thought he'd lost his ability to see due to the encephalitis (swelling of the brain). That day, God showed me that Stephen could see and hear.

That sign of hope gave me the strength to live another day. Watching Stephen fight to come back to life made me realize I had stopped fighting for my own.

That's when I started redefining what self-care really meant. It wasn't just spa days or vacations (although those are great too). It was **resting without guilt**. Saying no without over-explaining. Scheduling doctor appointments for myself—not just everyone else. Drinking water. Moving my body. Reconnecting with God, even if only for five quiet minutes before the sun came up.

I started asking myself hard questions: What do I need? What do I enjoy? What fills me back up? Slowly, I began carving out space in my life that was just for me—and I noticed the difference almost immediately. I had more patience. More presence. More peace. Taking care of myself didn't make me less of a wife or mother—it made me more grounded, more joyful, and more available.

The world celebrates women who sacrifice, but rarely do we praise women who choose to preserve themselves. I've learned that burnout is not a badge of honor. And martyrdom is not my calling. God didn't call me to be everything to everyone. He called me to steward the vessel He gave me—mind, body, and soul.

Self-care isn't optional. It's foundational.

Reflection:

You are not required to set yourself on fire to keep others warm. True strength is found in balance—not burnout. When you care for yourself, you model to those around you that worthiness isn't tied to performance. It's okay to rest. It's okay to pause. It's okay to choose you.

Journal Prompt:

Think about a time when your faith was tested.

- What did you learn about yourself?
- What did you learn about God?
- How did that experience shape your relationship with Him?

Write a letter to your past self in that moment of fear, reminding you of what you couldn't see yet—that you were never alone.

CHAPTER 11

When My Faith Was All I Had

There were many nights I didn't think I would make it through. I felt buried under the weight of disappointment, fear, confusion, and pain. Watching my son fight for his life, watching my daughter wrestle with emotions I couldn't fix, and carrying the responsibility of keeping our family afloat, it broke me in places I didn't even know existed.

But even in the middle of that breaking, I could still hear God.

Not loudly. Not always clearly. But He never left.

There were moments in the ICU when I would whisper prayers through tears. I didn't have long, eloquent words. All I had was "Help me, God." And somehow, that was enough. The same God who parted the Red Sea and calmed the storm was sitting beside me in a hospital room. I couldn't see Him, but I could feel Him.

I remember one particular night; I sat in a chair beside my son's hospital bed. The chair felt hard and cold. The cushion was red and round. I'll never forget the smell that permeated the room from the hallway. It smelled like old blood mixed with bleach. I remember so clearly, because the smell from the bleach was so strong, it caused a burning sensation inside my nostrils.

The overhead speaker reported a trauma had just arrived in room 3. We were in room 5. I could hear them calling for different medications, and multiple people ran past our room a few times. It was so chaotic that night. The monitors beeped, and machines hummed in the background, and a few seconds later, the overhead speaker chimed, "Code Blue, Room 3. Code Blue, Room 3."

Being in nursing, I knew that this meant either the patient's heart stopped beating or they stopped breathing. I sat still—heart racing, thoughts spiraling—praying my son wasn't next. Then I heard it. That still small voice again: "Your son will be okay." Unfortunately, I'm not sure if the other patient survived or not. The curtains to our room were pulled and the door was shut by the staff. I prayed that the patient in room 3 survived. What I do know is Stephen remained stable throughout the hospital stay and after discharge.

That moment became my anchor. It reminded me that I wasn't walking alone. That my faith wasn't in vain. That God didn't promise an easy journey, but He promised He'd never leave me. And He hasn't.

In the darkest seasons, faith was all I had—and it was enough.

When bills piled up, God provided. When sleep was stolen by stress, God sustained me. When I didn't know how to parent through the pain, God whispered wisdom. Through it all, I've learned that faith isn't always about shouting hallelujah; it's sometimes the quiet trust in the middle of chaos.

Reflection:

Faith doesn't always make sense, but it always makes a way. In your darkest hour, hold on. Even when your hands feel weak, even when your tears won't stop, even when the answers don't come, God is still there. And when your faith is all you have, it is more than enough.

Journal Prompt:

Think about a season in your life when everything felt uncertain or overwhelming, yet something—faith, hope, or a quiet strength—carried you through.

- What did faith look like for you in that season? Was it loud and bold, or soft and still?
- Were there moments when you felt God's presence in unexpected ways?
- What helped you hold on when you felt like giving up?

Reflect on how your faith grew during that time and how it continues to sustain you today.

CHAPTER 12

STILL STANDING – THE BEAUTY IN BECOMING

There were times I didn't think I'd make it to this moment.

Not just moments of exhaustion or fear—but moments when I questioned whether the pain would ever ease, whether the purpose was worth the pressure, and whether my story was worth sharing at all.

But I kept going.

Not because I had all the answers. Not because I was unbreakable.
I kept going because something deep inside whispered, *"This can't be the end of your story."*
And it wasn't.

I remember sitting in the hospital hallway, my hands trembling, wondering if I had anything left to give. The walls felt like they were closing in, and I questioned everything—my strength, my faith, even my identity. But somehow, I took another breath. And then another.

Healing wasn't instant. Some days, it came through tears. Other days, through laughter.

Some days, I stood strong. Other days, I crawled.
But through every setback, every silent prayer, and every brave step forward—I became.

I became a woman who honors her scars without hiding them—where once I saw shame, I now see strength.
I became a mother who loves fiercely through fatigue—where once I questioned if I was enough, I now lead with grace.
I became a caregiver who knows her worth is not tied to her capacity—where once I measured myself by how much I could do, I now rest in who I am.
I became a child of God who has learned that even in brokenness, beauty remains—where once I asked, "Why me?" I now whisper, "Thank you for the becoming. Thank you for trusting me with such a special assignment."

This journey has taught me that thriving isn't about having a perfect life.
It's about rising—even when the odds say you shouldn't.
It's about loving—even when love hasn't always been easy.
It's about choosing joy—even in the face of grief.

I don't have all the answers.
But I have faith. I have fight. I have a story.
And if you're reading this, so do you.

So, if you're standing here, uncertain of your next step, know this:
You don't have to have it all figured out.
Becoming isn't a final destination—it's a sacred unfolding.
Keep going.
Not because you're unshaken, but because you're worthy of what's ahead.

Reflection:

Sometimes the greatest evidence of healing is simply that we're still here showing up, loving, learning, and choosing to grow.
You don't have to have every wound stitched up or every question answered to begin living again.
Thriving doesn't mean the pain never happened. It means you're no longer letting it define your identity.

You've carried heavy things. You've endured what others couldn't imagine.
You've cried in silence, whispered prayers in the dark, and kept going even when you didn't feel strong.
That's not weakness. That's resilience. That's grace in motion.

Still standing doesn't mean you're not still healing.
It just means you've decided not to give up.

The journey isn't about perfection. It's about becoming.
And if you're still standing, you're already proof that healing is possible.

Journal Prompt:

Take a moment to reflect on your journey:

- What parts of your story once felt too painful to speak aloud but now feel like a testimony?
- What have you learned about yourself that surprised you in the process of healing?
- In what ways are you "thriving through the unexpected" right now—even if it still feels messy?

CHAPTER 13

THE LEGACY I'M BUILDING

Legacy isn't built in the spotlight—it's forged in the quiet, sacred places where no one sees you sowing, sacrificing, or showing up when it's hardest.

I didn't set out to build a legacy. I was just trying to survive. But somewhere in the survival, I began laying bricks—through every act of love, every prayer whispered in the dark, every decision to rise again.

This book isn't just a collection of memories; it's a living blueprint of what it means to pour out purpose even when life pours on the pain.

I chose to tell my story not for sympathy, but for strength. I want my children—and anyone who ever doubted their value—to know this truth: **Your voice matters. Your journey matters. And your legacy is not determined by perfection, but by presence.**

My legacy is layered. It's in every G-Tube feeding I gave with shaking hands, every care plan I created when the system fell short, every tear I wiped, and every decision I made rooted in love instead of fear.

It's also in the laughter we shared at the kitchen table. In the way I still show up on days I feel invisible. In the truth I tell even when it's uncomfortable.

I'm not leaving behind a story of ease. I'm leaving behind a story of endurance. Of a woman who dared to turn sorrow into strength and setbacks into seeds.

This chapter of my life is not the end—it's the handoff. One day, someone will hold these pages, and I hope they don't just see me. I hope they see themselves.

May they see what it looks like to lead with faith. To serve with heart. To keep going—not because it's easy, but because it's worth it.

Reflection:

Legacy isn't just about what you leave behind; it's about what you build with every choice, every truth, and every act of love.
You don't have to wait until you have it all together to leave something meaningful.
Right now, in your ordinary moments, you're writing history for someone else's healing.

Journal Prompt:

Think deeply and honestly:

- What values are you modeling today that you want others to carry forward?

- Who has influenced your definition of legacy, and how are you expanding it?
- What quiet decisions have you made recently that reflect the kind of legacy you want to leave?

A LETTER TO YOU – THE STORY CONTINUES

Dear Reader,

If you've made it this far, thank you from the depths of my heart. Thank you for walking with me through every twist, turn, tear, and triumph. Writing this book wasn't easy. It was tender, raw, and at times, deeply painful. But it was necessary. It was my way of taking back the narrative, of using the pain I once thought would break me to instead breathe life into someone else.

Maybe you picked up this book because you're carrying something heavy. Maybe you're a parent, a caregiver, a survivor, or simply someone trying to find light in the dark. Whoever you are—**you matter. Your story matters.** And no matter how broken it feels right now, there is hope.

I didn't write this because I've figured it all out. I wrote it because I know what it means to cry in secret, to question your worth, and to keep going anyway. I wrote it because I've lived through moments that tried to silence me and chose, instead, to speak. To live. To love. To build something new.

And I want that for you, too.

What was once broken in me is now being rebuilt into something beautiful. This story isn't about perfection—it's about persistence. It's about finding meaning in the mess, and strength in the struggle. It's about knowing that even in the darkest moments, there is light—sometimes flickering, sometimes faint, but always there.

My life is proof that you can be shattered and still shine.
That you can lose everything and still find yourself.
That grief and joy can live in the same room.
That with faith, nothing is wasted.

So, if you're still in the middle of your storm—**keep going.**
If you feel unseen—**know that you are deeply valued.**
And if you're wondering whether you can make it—**let me be your reminder that yes, you absolutely can.**

To every mother, caregiver, friend, or reader who saw themselves in these pages—thank you. Thank you for letting me share my story with you. I pray that something here reminded you that you are not alone, and that healing is possible—even if it doesn't look like what you expected.

This isn't the end. It's the beginning.
The beginning of healing.
The beginning of legacy.
The beginning of a life that thrives—not in spite of pain, but because you dared to rise through it.

Let's continue to rise, to fight, to love, and to live—fully and boldly.

Because we're not just surviving anymore.

We're *thriving.*

With love,

Latrina

Reflection:

You've just finished reading a story of heartbreak, healing, and becoming.
But your story isn't over.
Right now, you have the power to choose what comes next.
Whether you're still in the middle or just beginning, your presence matters.

You've survived what you thought might break you—and that means there is strength in you still unfolding.

Journal Prompt:

- What part of my story resonated most deeply with your own life?
- In what ways have you surprised yourself with your own strength or growth?
- What would it mean for you to move from simply surviving to truly thriving?
- If you wrote a letter to your future self today, what truth or encouragement would you want to include?

ACKNOWLEDGMENTS

Behind every story told is a circle of people who made the telling possible.

To God, my anchor—thank You for being the constant in my chaos, the peace in my pain, and the light in every dark place. When life felt unbearable and I didn't have the strength to stand, You carried me. Every chapter of this book is laced with Your grace. I didn't write this alone—You were with me in every sentence, every tear, every breakthrough. Thank You for never letting go, even when I wanted to give up.

To my son—you are the heartbeat behind these pages. Your resilience, your joy, your quiet strength, and your ability to smile in the face of adversity have shaped me more than you'll ever know. Watching you fight battles you didn't ask for—and doing it with such grace—has given me a deeper understanding of courage. You inspire me to keep going, to keep believing, and to keep writing. You are my why. I love you.

To my husband—thank you for standing beside me through the storms I didn't have words for. Your quiet strength, unwavering love, and ability to hold space for my healing have meant more than I could ever express. When I was tired, you gave me rest. When I doubted myself, you reminded me of who I am. You've been my safe place—and for that, I'm forever grateful. I love you.

To my daughter—thank you for loving me through my imperfections. For seeing me not just as your mother, but as a woman learning to navigate grief, purpose, and self-discovery. Your patience, your presence, and your willingness to walk this journey with me—even when it wasn't easy—mean the world to me. You are one of my greatest gifts. I see you. I thank you. I love you.

To my family and close friends—thank you for your prayers, hugs, and encouragement when I couldn't see the next step.

To the special needs community and every caregiver walking through the unexpected—you are not alone. This book is for us.

To Kemone and Rhiann at THP Editing Service (@THPeditingServc)—thank you for walking this journey with me. Your insight, patience, and thoughtful feedback helped me shape this story in a way that honored both the pain and the purpose behind every word. You treated my manuscript with care and intention, and I'm so grateful for your heart, your time, and your expertise.

To Lauren Zoucha—thank you for capturing more than just images. You captured emotion, strength, and the quiet resilience behind our smile. Your work gave this book a visual heartbeat, and I'm so thankful for your creative eye and your gentle spirit.

AUTHOR'S NOTE

This book was never meant to be a fairytale. It was meant to be real.

Real faith.
Real pain.
Real healing.
Real hope.

If you've walked through deep waters, I hope you found a piece of yourself in these pages.
If you're just beginning your journey, I hope you found the strength to take your next step.

Every sentence was written with you in mind.
You are not alone, and you never were.
This isn't just my story; it's a reminder that we all carry something sacred.

Thank you for letting me share my truth. I pray you carry it forward with grace.

My Favorite Scripture:

"Trust in the Lord with all your heart
and lean not on your own understanding;
in all your ways submit to Him,
and He will make your paths straight."
— *Proverbs 3:5–6 (NIV)*

ABOUT THE AUTHOR

Latrina Lenoir is a devoted mother, nurse practitioner, and advocate for families navigating life after unexpected trials. After her son became permanently disabled following a sudden illness, Latrina began sharing her story to bring light, strength, and hope to other caregivers, mothers, and women learning to thrive through heartbreak.

With a voice rooted in faith and authenticity, she empowers others to rise, rebuild, and rediscover their purpose—one chapter at a time.

When she's not writing, Latrina creates faith-based content on YouTube and serves as a mentor for women walking through life's deepest valleys.

INVITATION TO CONNECT

Your story matters—and it deserves to be heard.

If this book spoke to you, encouraged you, or helped you feel seen, I would love to hear from you. Your words remind me why I keep sharing mine.

Let's continue walking this journey together.
Let's keep rising, even when it's hard.
Let's keep thriving—through every unexpected turn.

You can connect with me at:

info@latrinalenoir.com

Instagram: Iamlatrinalenoir

YouTube: @ThrivewithLatrina

Facebook Group: *The Sunflower Circle*

You were never meant to do this alone.
I'm cheering for you—every step of the way.

www.ingramcontent.com/pod-product-compliance
Lightning Source LLC
LaVergne TN
LVHW022005200926
848481LV00007B/2249